The Busy Mom Cookbook

15-Minute Homemade Express Dinners When You're Just Too Busy (40 Recipes Included)!

by Olivia Rogers

Copyright © 2018 By Olivia Rogers
All rights reserved. No part of this book may be reproduced in any form without permission in writing from the author. No part of this publication may be reproduced or transmitted in any form or by any means, mechanic, electronic, photocopying, recording, by any storage or retrieval system, or transmitted by email without the permission in writing from the author and publisher.
For information regarding permissions write to author at Olivia@TheMenuAtHome.com
Reviewers may quote brief passages in review.

Please note that credit for the images used in this book go to the respective owners. You can view this at:
TheMenuAtHome.com/image-list

Olivia Rogers
TheMenuAtHome.com

Table of Contents

Introduction _____ 5
1. Pesto Chicken Pasta _____ 6
2. Lamb Burgers _____ 9
3. Salmon & Slaw _____ 11
4. Pesto Halibut _____ 13
5. Blackened Chicken with Quinoa Salad _____ 15
6. Basil Prosciutto Pizza _____ 19
7. Broiler Salmon with Tomatoes _____ 21
8. Almond Crusted Cod _____ 23
9. Caprese Melt _____ 25
10. Ricotta Fritters with Salad _____ 27
11. Lentil Paneer Salad _____ 30
12. Chicken Sausage Stew _____ 32
13. Salad Pizzas _____ 34
14. Crab Couscous _____ 36
15. Quick Steak Sauté _____ 39
16. Hearty Chicken Soup _____ 41
17. Portobello Burgers _____ 43
18. Mushroom Soup _____ 45
19. Spicy Garlic Prawns _____ 48
20. Buffalo Chicken Burgers _____ 50
21. Quick Falafels _____ 52
22. Veggie Chili with Salad _____ 54
23. Fried Rice and Eggs _____ 57

24. Buttermilk Chicken Salad	59
25. Portobello Mushroom Salad	61
26. Beef Kofta on Rice	63
27. Lemon Tuna Pasta	66
28. Ravioli Zucchini Sauté	68
29. Almond Kale Salad	70
30. Stuffed Quesadillas	72
31. Pork Tofu Stir-Fry	74
32. Tuna Bean Salad	76
33. Tarragon Chicken	78
34. Spaghetti with Fresh Tomato Sauce and Basil Leaves	80
35. Sea Bream Baked with Rosemary and Lemon	82
36. Brown Onion and Garlic Soup with Sour Cream	84
37. Pressure Cooker Chicken with Orange	86
38. Thai Seafood Curry with Egg Noodles	88
39. Baked Pizza Rolls	91
40. Super Fast Pizza	93
Final Words	95
Disclaimer	97

Introduction

Cooking dinner every night is not only exhausting, it's a real challenge, especially after a long day at work. This is when nobody wants to spend hours slaving over a hot stove, unfortunately, for many of us, this usually means giving in to the temptation of having fast food or frozen TV dinners.

These options are usually unhealthy and expensive, with the cost of eating this way, adding up quickly and the possibility of causing our overall health to decline. This book offers an easy way to help you make quick, effortless meals in under 15 minutes. Meals that taste better and are more nutritious than TV dinners and fast food take out. Delicious meals that will save you money and your health.

With the help and ideas in this book you will be able to create a huge variety of nutritious and scrumptious meals for the whole family without having to spend more than 15 minutes cooking. Every recipe in this book can be done in a matter of minutes AND they are all created to give meals that are packed with the nutrients you and your family need each day!

1. Pesto Chicken Pasta

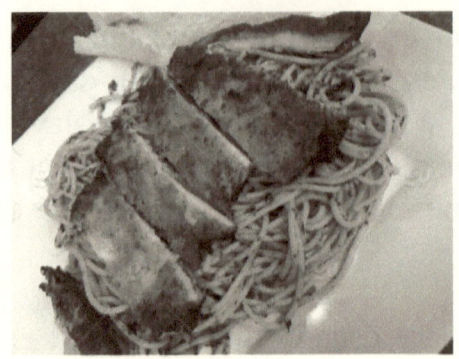

Serves 2 people

Pesto is a simple, healthy way to add a flavorful punch to this simple dish.

Ingredients

- 1 lb. of Skinless Chicken Breasts
- 1 tsp. of Fennel Seeds
- 2 sprigs of Rosemary
- 4 Tbsps. of Olive Oil (divided)
- 5 cloves of Garlic (crushed)
- 2 Red Chilies
- 8 Cherry Tomatoes (halved)

- ½ a lb. of Green Beans

- 1 bunch of Basil

- 2-3 handfuls of Blanched Almonds

- ¼ cup of Grated Parmesan

- 1 Lemon

- ½ lb. of Pasta (any)

- ½ lb. of Fresh Spinach

Method

1. Toss the chicken and fennel seeds, rosemary, salt, and pepper together on a large sheet of parchment paper. Fold the paper to cover and seal the chicken. Then flatten the chicken with a rolling pin until it becomes thin.

2. Place the flattened chicken pieces in a pan over a high heat with 2 tablespoons oil. Add the chilies and garlic. Cook each side for about 3-4 minutes. Place the green beans in a casserole dish and cover with pre-boiled salt water. Put the lid on and simmer them for 6 minutes over medium heat.

3. Remove stalks from the basil leaves and place them in a blender or food processor with the almonds, Parmesan, 2 tablespoons of oil, and the lemon juice. Pulse the

mixture a few times, then add the cooked garlic from the pan to this mixture. Then process it, just until the mixture becomes evenly mixed. If necessary, add a few tablespoons of salt water from the beans to help create a smooth consistency and season with a little more salt and pepper to taste.

4. Add the pasta to the green beans and let them cook a few minutes until "al dente". Add the tomatoes to the chicken and toss to mix. Stir the spinach into the pasta and green beans. Remove 1 cup of cooking water and set it aside. Drain the rest.

5. Combine the pasta, beans, spinach, and pesto mixture in the casserole dish until well mixed. If necessary, add a few tablespoons of cooking water to give a smoother texture. Slice the chicken so that you have 4 pieces.

6. To serve, divide the pasta mixture onto 2 plates, place the chicken on top and garnish with the tomatoes, and chilies.

2. Lamb Burgers

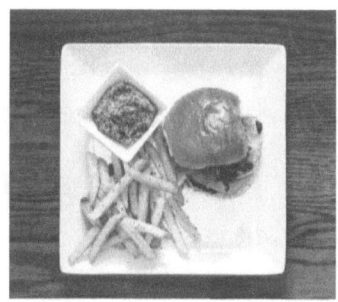

Serves 4 people

The combination of lamb and hummus, puts a delicious twist on the classic burger recipe.

Ingredients

- 1 lb. of Ground Lamb

- 1/3 of a cup of Tomato Relish

- 4 Buns (toasted)

- ¼ of a cup of Hummus

- 2-3 handfuls of Fresh Spinach

- ½ a cup of Fire-Roasted Peppers (sliced)

- ½ a cup of Crumbled Feta

Method

1. Set your grill to a medium to high heat. In a bowl, mix together the ground lamb and relish, then divide them into 4 and shape each one into a patty.

2. Cook the patties on the grill for 4 minutes on each side and toast the buns.

3. Spread the hummus on your hot toasted buns, then place the spinach, patties, feta, and peppers on top of the hummus and serve with extra pesto and seasoned fries.

3. Salmon & Slaw

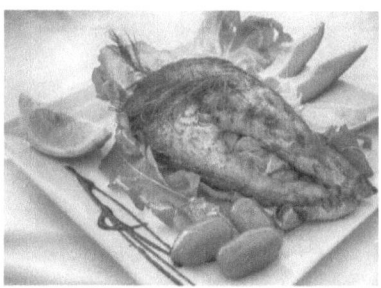

Serves 2 people

Whip up this elegant and satisfying salmon dinner in just 15 minutes.

Ingredients

- 1 ¼ lbs. of Skinless Salmon Fillets (4 pieces)
- 1 tsp of Olive Oil
- 6 cups of Bok Choy (thinly sliced) or Rocket lettuce
- 1 Red Apple (diced)
- 1 tomato, cut in wedges
- 4 Scallions (thinly sliced)
- 1/3 of a cup of Plain Greek Yogurt
- 2 Tbsps. of Fresh Squeezed Lemon Juice

- Salt & Pepper to taste

Method

1. Place the oil in a large skillet on a medium to high heat. Rub the salmon fillets with ¼ tsp each of salt and pepper, then cook them in the skillet for 2-3 minutes per side.

2. In a bowl, toss together the Bok Choy or rocket lettuce, apple, tomato and scallions. Mix in the yogurt, lemon juice, and remaining salt and pepper. Serve this next to the salmon.

4. Pesto Halibut

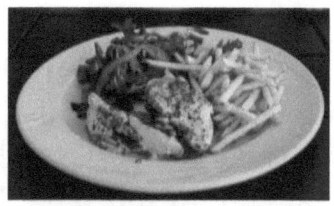

Makes enough for 4 people

Tomato and pesto add rich dimensions of flavor to this halibut dinner.

Ingredients

- 2 Garlic Cloves
- 2 Tbsps. of Toasted Almonds
- 4 cups of Kale (torn)
- ½ a cup (+ 1 Tbsp.) of Olive Oil (divided)
- ¼ of a cup of Grated Parmesan
- 1-2 Tbsps. of Fresh Squeezed Lemon Juice
- ¾ of a tsp of Salt (divided)
- ¾ of a tsp of Pepper (divided)
- 4 Halibut Fillets

- 1 lb. of Cherry Tomatoes (halved)

Method

1. Preheat your oven to 400°F. Pulse together in a food processor or blender the garlic and nuts. Add 2 cups of kale, ½ a cup of oil, the lemon juice, and Parmesan. Pulse this mixture until it's thoroughly mixed.

2. Add the remaining kale with ½ a tsp each of salt and pepper, then process this mixture until thoroughly blended.

3. Heat 1 tablespoon oil in a skillet over medium to high heat. Add the halibut and cook it for 2-3 minutes on one side only. Remove the skillet from the heat and turn the halibut over. Add the tomatoes and sprinkle them with the remaining salt and pepper. Bake it in your preheated oven for 7-10 minutes.

4. Top the Halibut fillets with the fresh kale pesto and serve it with a green leafy salad and fries.

5. Blackened Chicken with Quinoa Salad

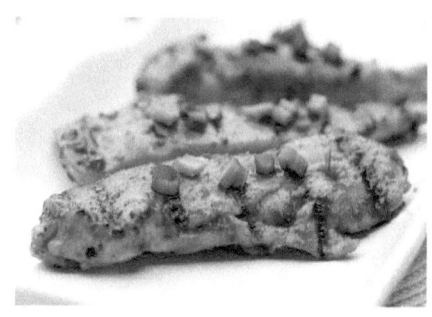

Makes 4 servings

Put these lovely chicken breasts together with quinoa, spinach cilantro and mint for a quick, hearty and satisfying salad, ideal for lunch or dinner.

Ingredients

- 1 ½ cups of Quinoa
- 1 Red Chili
- 3-4 handfuls of Fresh Spinach
- 4 Spring Onions
- 1 bunch of Fresh Cilantro
- 1 bunch of Fresh Mint
- 1 large Mango (peeled, chopped)

- 2 Limes
- 1 Avocado (peeled and sliced)
- 4 Tbsps. of Olive Oil (divided)
- ¼ of a cup of Crumbled Feta
- 1 Punnet of Cress
- 1 lb. of Skinless Chicken Breasts
- 1 tsp of Ground Allspice
- 2 Bell Peppers (sliced)
- 4 Tbsps. of Plain Greek Yogurt

Method

1. Place a saucepan on a medium to high heat with 3 cups of water, enough to completely submerge the Quinoa. When the water is boiling, add 1 tsp of sea salt and the quinoa, then cook it for 12 minutes uncovered on a medium heat. The liquid should almost, all, be absorbed.

2. In a processor or blender, pulse together the spinach, spring onions, cilantro, chili, and mint leaves until they are finely chopped.

3. Place the allspice, paprika, salt and pepper on a large sheet of parchment paper and toss the chicken in it to completely cover. Then fold the paper so it covers the chicken. Roll or beat the chicken out so it becomes thin, allowing it to cook quickly retaining its tenderness and moisture.

4. Place 1 Tbsp of oil in a pan on high heat, when it is hot, place in the chicken. Turn it after 3-4 minutes and allow the skin to become blackened.

5. Remove the chicken from the pan and add the peppers with a little more oil and cook them until they become softened.

6. After 12 minutes, drain and rinse the quinoa. Toss it together with the spinach mixture and the juice from the limes as well as the remaining oil ensuring it is well mixed. Taste it to check the seasoning and add salt and pepper if necessary.

7. Sprinkle the chopped mango and peppers over the quinoa. Top this with avocado slices. Slice up chicken and place it on top of quinoa. Sprinkle on the feta crumbles, cilantro, and cress. Serve with a dollop of yogurt.

Read This FIRST - 100% FREE BONUS

FOR A LIMITED TIME ONLY – Get Olivia's best-selling book *"The #1 Cookbook: Over 170+ of the Most Popular Recipes Across 7 Different Cuisines!"* absolutely FREE!

Readers have absolutely loved this book because of the wide variety of recipes. It is highly recommended you check these recipes out and see what you can add to your home menu!

Once again, as a big thank-you for downloading this book, I'd like to offer it to you *100% FREE for a LIMITED TIME ONLY!*

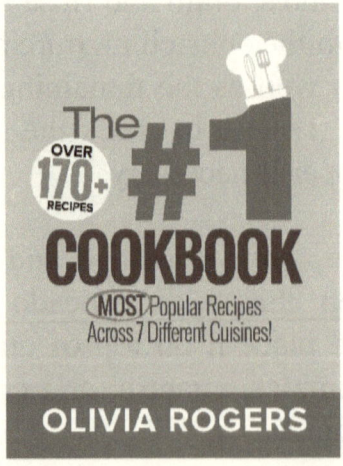

Get your free copy at:

TheMenuAtHome.com/Bonus

6. Basil Prosciutto Pizza

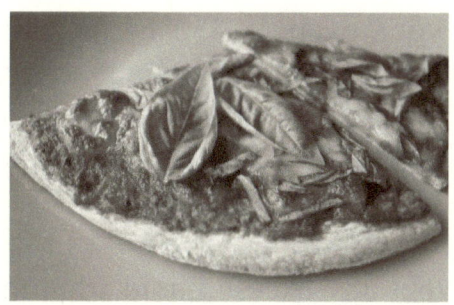

Serves 2 people

This quick pizza recipe makes a delicious and healthy dinner that the whole family will love.

Ingredients

- ½ a lb. of Small Tomatoes (halved)

- ½ a lb. of Fresh Spinach

- 2 large pieces Flat Bread

- ½ a lb. of Grated Mozzarella

- ½ a lb. of Ricotta

- ¼ of a cup of Basil, Cashew & Parmesan Dip

- 6 slices of Prosciutto

Method

1. Preheat your oven to 450°F. In a bowl, steep the spinach for 1 minute in boiling water, then drain it and set it aside. Place the bread on a baking sheet lined with parchment paper. Then spread the ricotta on top.

2. Squeeze out any excess liquid from the spinach and arrange it on top of the bread. Add the tomato, mozzarella, and prosciutto.

3. Bake the pizzas for 5 minutes on a high heat in a pre-heated oven or under a broiler. Spoon on the basil dip. Then season it to taste with pepper before serving.

7. Broiler Salmon with Tomatoes

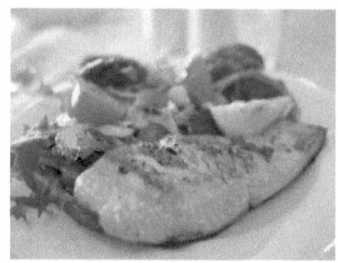

Makes 4 servings

This juicy tomato and salmon dish pairs perfectly with a quinoa salad. The trick is to only cook the salmon to rear or medium rare and not to overcook it.

Ingredients

- 4 (6oz.) pieces of Skinless Salmon Fillets
- 4 Tomatoes (halved)
- 2 Tbsps. of Olive Oil
- ½ a tsp of Paprika
- 8 Sprigs of Thyme
- 4 Garlic Cloves (sliced)
- Salt & Pepper to taste

Method

1. Heat your broiler to a medium to high heat. Place the tomatoes and salmon in a broiler-safe pan and drizzle them liberally with oil.

2. Season them with salt and pepper to taste and also sprinkle on the paprika, thyme, and garlic. Broil the fillets for 8-10 minutes. Arrange on a plate with the salad of your choice.

8. Almond Crusted Cod

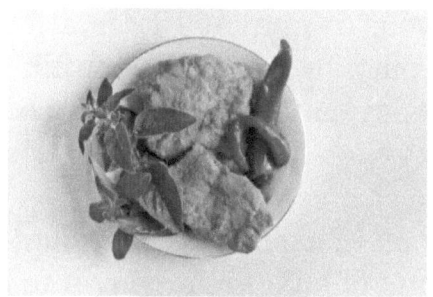

Makes 2 servings

Impress your guests with this quick, elegant and tasty cod dinner.

Ingredients

- 1 Whole Grain English Muffin (torn into pieces)
- ¼ of a cup of Sliced Almonds
- 4 tsp of Olive Oil
- 1 tsp of Thyme
- Salt & Pepper to taste
- 4 (6oz.) pieces of Skinless Cod
- 2 tsp of Mayonnaise

Method

1. Preheat your oven to 400°F. In a food processor or blender, pulse together the muffin pieces, thyme, and almonds until the mixture becomes coarsely blended.

2. Place the oil in a pan over a medium-high heat, then add the crumb mixture, tossing it to evenly coat the crumbs in the oil. Cook this mixture for 3 minutes, stirring occasionally.

3. Arrange the cod on a baking sheet lined with parchment paper. Spread the mayonnaise evenly over each piece. Then spread the crumb mixture evenly over top side, pressing it down lightly.

4. Bake the cod for about 8 minutes and serve with your favorite salad.

9. Caprese Melt

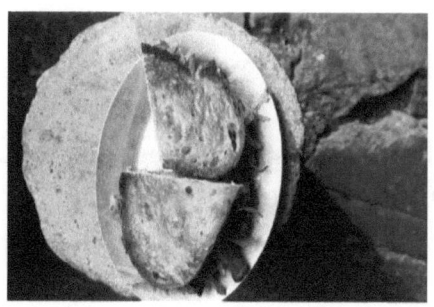

Serves 2 people

This recipe combines the classic grilled cheese with a Caprese salad.

Ingredients

- 6 slices of Sourdough Bread
- 1-2 Tbsps. of Olive Oil
- 15 Fresh Basil Leaves
- 2 large Tomatoes (sliced)
- 4 oz. of Fresh Mozzarella (sliced)
- Salt & Pepper to taste

Method

1. Brush one side of each slice of the bread with olive oil. Place 3 of slices oil side up, on a baking sheet. Layer on the bread the basil, tomato, and mozzarella.

2. Season them with salt and pepper to taste, then place the remaining bread on top. Broil the sandwiches 2-3 minutes, turning them once. Then serve hot.

10. Ricotta Fritters with Salad

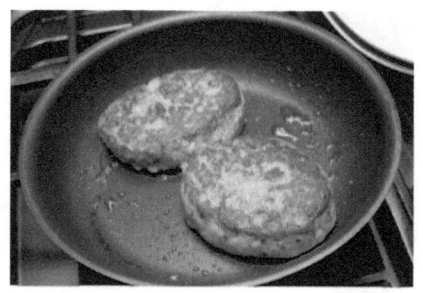

Enough for 4 servings

This effortless dish creates an unforgettable flavor combination with it's mushroom, chili, and mint.

Ingredients

- 1-2 oz. of Dried Porcini Mushrooms
- 4 Anchovy Fillets
- 1 Dried Red Chili
- 2 Garlic Cloves
- 3 cups of Tomato Paste
- 8 Black Olives
- 1 large Egg
- 2 cups of Ricotta

- 2 tsp of Nutmeg

- 2 Lemons (divided)

- 2-3 oz. of Parmesan

- 1 Tbsp. of Flour

- Olive Oil

- Balsamic Vinegar

- 1 lb. of Zucchini

- 1 Fresh Red Chili

- ½ a bunch of Fresh Mint (chopped)

- ½ a bunch of Fresh Basil (chopped)

Method

1. Place the mushrooms to soak and soften in a cup of hot water. In a bowl, beat together until combined the egg, ricotta, nutmeg, lemon zest, and Parmesan, then whisk in the flour.

2. Heat 1 tablespoon of oil in a pan on medium heat. Spoon the egg mixture into the hot pan in 8 separate dollops to create the fritters.

3. Place 1 Tbsp of the oil into a casserole dish or saucepan on a low heat and add the anchovies, stir in the dried chili and crushed garlic.

4. Drain and chop the mushrooms, reserving half of the water. Add the mushrooms, tomato paste and reserved water to the anchovy mixture. Season this with salt and pepper to taste. Bring the mixture to a low simmer and add the olives and basil.

5. Coarsely chop the zucchini in a food processor. Then toss them with salt, pepper, 1 tablespoon of oil, and the juice from 1 lemon, add the fresh chili and mint. Then toss all of these together to combine.

6. Place a little of the sauce on each serving plate, then place the fritters on top of the sauce. Drizzle balsamic over the top and serve them with the zucchini salad and lemon wedges.

11. Lentil Paneer Salad

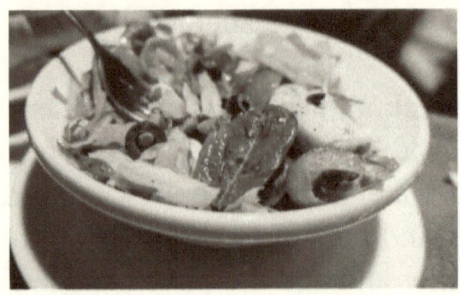

Makes 2 servings

Lentils and paneer create a hearty salad with the bold flavors reminiscent of Indian cuisine.

Ingredients

- 1 lb. of Paneer (thinly sliced)

- 1 tsp of Curry Powder (divided)

- 1/3 of a cup of Olive Oil

- 1 Onion (thinly sliced)

- 1 Red Bell Pepper (thinly sliced)

- 2 Garlic Cloves (minced)

- 1 lb. of canned Brown Lentils (drained)

- 2 Tbsps. of Mango Chutney

- 1 Tbsp of sliced Black Olives
- 1 Tbsp. of Apple Cider Vinegar
- 1 cup of Fresh Spinach
- Naan and plain Greek Yogurt to serve

Method

1. Toss together the Paneer ½ a tsp of curry powder and salt to taste in a bowl. Place 1 Tbsp of oil in a pan on a medium to high heat and cook the Paneer for 2-3 minutes, turning occasionally. Drain it on paper towels to remove the excess oil, then set it aside.

2. Add another Tbsp of oil to the pan and cook the onion for 3-4 minutes, stirring frequently. Add the peppers and garlic, and continue cooking them for 2-3 minutes, stirring occasionally. Add the lentils and remaining curry powder and cook the mixture for a further 1-2 minutes, stirring constantly. Remove it from the heat and set it aside.

3. In a small bowl, combine the vinegar, chutney, 2 Tbsp of oil, with the salt and pepper to taste to form the dressing. Combine the lentil mixture, spinach, and Paneer together and drizzle the dressing over the top. Serve it with naan and yogurt.

12. Chicken Sausage Stew

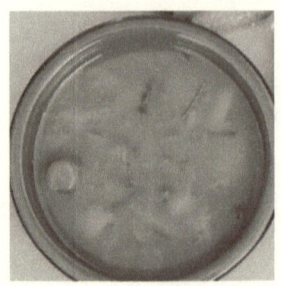

Enough for 4 servings

This quick stew recipe is guaranteed to leave everyone feeling full and satisfied.

Ingredients

- 1 Tbsp. of Olive Oil

- 1 (12oz.) package of Cooked Chicken Sausage (sliced)

- 1 (19oz.) can of White Beans (drained)

- 1 (14.5oz.) can of Chicken Broth

- 1 (14.5oz.) can of Diced Tomatoes

- 1 bunch of Kale (torn)

- Salt & Pepper to taste

- 1 loaf of Crusty Bread to serve

Method

1. Heat the oil in a large pot over a medium heat. Add the sausage, cooking it for 2-3 minutes, stirring occasionally. Add the garlic and cook a further 2 minutes, stirring often.

2. Add the broth, tomatoes (with liquid), and the beans. Bring the soup to the boil, then add the kale, with salt and pepper to taste. Reduce the heat to a simmer and stir it until the kale is wilted (2-3 minutes). Serve with the bread.

13. Salad Pizzas

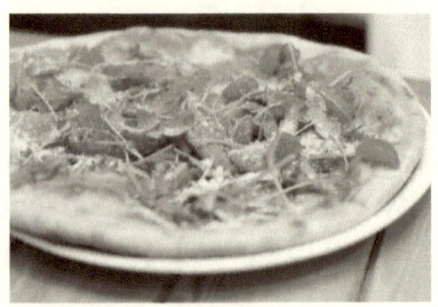

Makes 4 Pizzas

These pizzas are topped with fresh salad ingredients for a healthy and delicious recipe with amazing texture combinations.

Ingredients

- 4 Pitas
- 2 Garlic Cloves (minced)
- 1 cup of Grated Mozzarella
- ½ a cup of sliced Onion
- 1 Tbsp. of Cider Vinegar
- 1 tsp of Crushed Red Pepper Flakes
- 1 cup of Grape Tomatoes (quartered)

- ¼ of a cup of Kalamata Olives (chopped)

- 2 Tbsps. of Basil

- 4 cups of fresh Salad Greens

Method

1. Preheat your oven to 475°F and place the pitas on a lightly oiled baking sheet. Spread the minced garlic evenly across each pita and then sprinkle them with mozzarella. Divide the onion slices evenly among each of the pita. Bake them for 8 minutes.

2. In a bowl, whisk together the oil, vinegar, and pepper. Stir in the tomatoes, basil, and olives. Add the salad greens and toss the salad to coat it evenly. Place the salad mixture on top of each pita and serve.

14. Crab Couscous

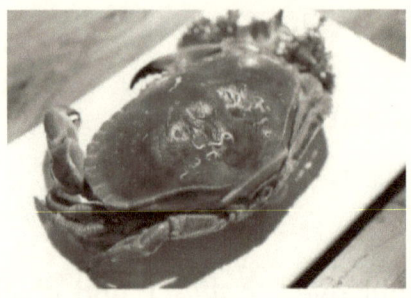

To make 4 portions

Crab stuffed pastries make this couscous dinner absolutely irresistible.

Ingredients

- 1-2 Preserved Lemons (chopped)

- 2 Spring Onions (chopped)

- ½ a bunch of Fresh Cilantro (chopped)

- 1 lb. of Crabmeat

- 2 tsp of Harissa (plus extra)

- 4 large sheets of Filo Pastry

- Olive Oil

- ½ a tsp of Caraway Seeds

- ¾ of a cup of Couscous

- 1 (6oz.) can of Tomato Paste

- ½ a Fennel Bulb (chopped)

- ½ a bunch of Fresh Mint (chopped)

- 1 ½ Lemons (divided)

- 1 Pomegranate (seeds removed)

- 1 large Tomato (grated)

- 1 (2") piece of Ginger (grated)

- Plain Greek Yogurt to serve

Method

1. In a bowl, mix together the crabmeat, harissa, preserved lemons, spring onions, and cilantro. Divide the crab mixture evenly into 4 and place it on each pastry sheet. Press your thumb in the middle of the crab mixture to leave a space, then fold the pastry until it is about the size of a deck of cards.

2. Heat 1 tablespoon of oil in a large pan on medium heat. Add the crab pastries and cook them until they are golden brown on both sides. Add the caraway seeds to the pan (around the pastries) and cook for 1

minute. Scoop the seeds into a salad bowl and remove the pastries, setting them aside.

3. Put the couscous in a pot with 1¾ cups of water; add the tomato paste and a dash of salt. Cover it and allow it to simmer for 12 minutes.

4. In the bowl with the caraway seeds, add and toss together the fennel, mint, and the juice of 1 lemon. Add a tablespoon of olive oil, salt and pepper to taste and toss these to combine.

5. Combine the tomato and ginger in a bowl with salt and pepper to taste. Add the juice from ½ a lemon and 1 tablespoon of olive oil. Mix these well together.

6. Stir the couscous to fluff it up, then pour it onto a platter, create a large dent in the middle of the pile. Fill the center with the mint mixture and sprinkle the pomegranate seeds on top. Serve this alongside the crab pastries with a dollop of yogurt and the tomato-ginger mixture.

15. Quick Steak Sauté

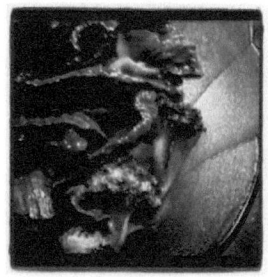

Serves 2 people

Fry up this scrumptious steak dinner in a matter of minutes.

Ingredients

- 3 bunches of Broccoli (chopped)
- 2 Tbsps. of Olive Oil
- 1 Fresh Red Chili (chopped)
- 2 Garlic Cloves (crushed)
- 2 Anchovy Fillets (chopped)
- 1 lb. of canned White Beans (drained)
- 12 thin pieces of Steak
- 2 Tbsps. of Lemon Juice

Method

1. Steam the broccoli in a double boiler for 2 minutes, then drain and rinse it with cold water to refresh and retain its color.

2. Heat 1 Tbsp of the oil in a pan over a medium heat. Add to this the anchovy, garlic, and chili. Cook these for 1 minute, stirring constantly, then add the broccoli, salt and pepper to taste. Cook this mixture for 3 minutes, stirring occasionally.

3. Add the white beans and continue cooking for 1-2 minutes, stirring often. Reduce the heat to the lowest setting to keep it warm.

4. Heat the remaining oil in another pan on a high heat. Rub the steaks with salt and pepper and cook each one for 1 to 2 minutes, turning occasionally. Remove them from the heat and set the steaks aside.

5. Add the lemon juice to the oil in the pan and scrape the bottom of the pan with wooden spoon for about 30 seconds (deglazing). Transfer lemon juice and oil to a bowl. Place 3 steaks on each plate. Top with bean mixture and drizzle with lemon-oil mixture from the pan.

16. Hearty Chicken Soup

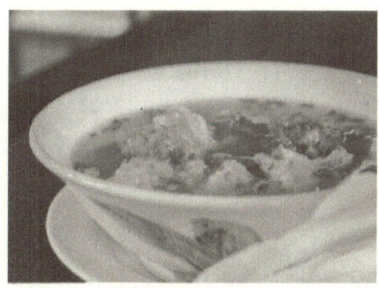

Makes 4 servings

Chicken, beans and sour cream combine for a soup that is simply perfect.

Ingredients

- 1 (12oz.) jar of Salsa Verde
- 3 cups of cooked Diced Chicken
- 1 (15oz.) can of White Beans (drained)
- 3 cups of Chicken Broth or Stock
- 1 tsp of Ground Cumin
- 2 Green Onions (chopped)
- ½ a cup of Sour Cream
- Tortilla Chips

Method

1. Heat the salsa in a large pot on medium-high heat for 2 minutes. Add the broth, beans, chicken, and cumin. Bring this to the boil, then reduce the heat to a medium simmer.

2. Cook the soup for about 10 minutes, stirring occasionally. Divide the soup into 4 serving bowls and top each with onions, tortilla chips, and sour cream.

17. Portobello Burgers

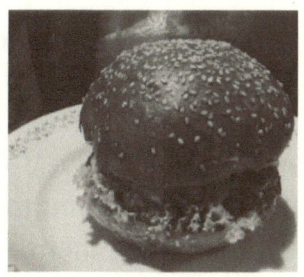

Makes 4 burgers

Soft, delicious Portobello mushroom tops are used instead of beef patties in this delicious burger recipe.

Ingredients

- 2 tsp of Olive Oil

- 4 large Portobello Tops

- 2-3 Garlic Cloves (minced)

- ¼ of a cup of Crumbled Gorgonzola

- 4 Tbsps. of Mayonnaise

- 4 Burger Buns

- 2 cups of Arugula

- ½ a cup of Bottled Roasted Red Bell Peppers

- Lettuce leaves

- Salt & Pepper to taste

Method

1. Heat the oil in a large pan on a medium-heat and cut the buns in half, then toast them.

2. Sprinkle salt and pepper over the mushrooms and then saute them in the pan, stirring constantly and turning once, if needed, add a Tbsp of fresh water.

3. After about 4 minutes, add the garlic and cook another 30 seconds, stirring constantly, then remove this mixture from the heat.

4. In a bowl, mix together the cheese and mayonnaise. Place a lettuce leaf on the bottom slice of each toasted bun, then spread on the cheese mixture. Divide the arugula and peppers evenly amongst each bun. Place 1 mushroom on top of each and cover them with the top slice of bun and serve.

18. Mushroom Soup

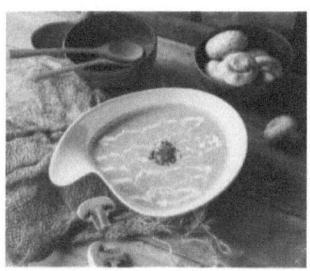

Makes 4 generous servings

This mushroom soup is beautifully paired with the apple walnut toasts found in this recipe.

Ingredients

- 2 Onions (thinly sliced)
- 1 cube of Chicken Stock
- ½ a bunch of Fresh Thyme (chopped)
- 2 Garlic Cloves (minced)
- 1 Garlic Clove (halved)
- 4 large Portobello Mushrooms
- ½ a cup of Basmati Rice
- 1 Tbsp. of Cream

- 8 Chestnut Mushrooms

- 1 loaf of Ciabatta (cut into 4 slices)

- 1 Apple (grated)

- ½ a bunch of Fresh Parsley (chopped)

- 1 Lemon

- 3-4 oz. of Blue Cheese

- 1 handful of Walnuts

- 1 Quart of boiling Water

- Olive Oil as needed

Method

1. Heat 2 tablespoons oil in a large pan on medium heat. Add the onions and saute them for 2 minutes. Crumble in the cube of chicken stock and add a pinch of salt and pepper, then stir in the thyme and minced garlic.

2. While the onions are cooking, remove the stems from the chestnut mushrooms and place the tops on a griddle over high heat, charring both sides, then put them to the side.

3. Toss the chestnut mushroom stems with the onions, add the Portobello mushrooms and the rice cooking these for 2 minutes, stirring constantly.

4. Pour in 1 quart of boiling water, cover it and allow it to boil a few minutes. Place the ciabatta on griddle pan. Char both sides. Rub each side with the halved garlic.

5. In a bowl, mix the apple, parsley, and lemon juice. Divide the chestnut mushrooms among the ciabatta slices. Crumble blue cheese over the tops and sprinkle them with the walnuts. Place the toast on a prepared grill on high heat until cheese just melts.

6. Use a stick blender to puree the mushroom and rice mixture until it's smooth, then stir in the cream. Spread the apple mixture on top of the ciabatta toast and serve it alongside the mushroom soup.

19. Spicy Garlic Prawns

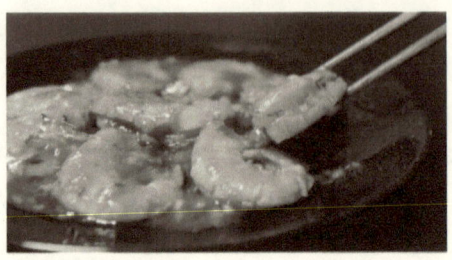

To serve 4 people

This recipe is one of the easiest and tastiest ways to enjoy a plate of prawns.

Ingredients

- 2lbs of fresh or frozen Prawns (shelled)
- 6 Tbsps. of Butter
- 2 Tbsps. of Olive Oil
- 4 Garlic Cloves (thinly sliced)
- 2 Fresh Red Chilies
- 2 Tbsps. of Fresh Lemon Juice
- 3 tsp of Lemon Zest
- ¼ of a cup of Fresh Cilantro (chopped)

- Arugula to serve

- Grilled Crusty Bread (brushed with oil) to serve

Method

1. Heat the butter and oil in a large pan over a medium-high heat. Stir in the garlic and chilies. Cook 1 minute, stirring constantly. Add the prawns with salt and pepper to taste.

2. Cook the prawns only for 3-4 minutes (do not over cook). Add the cilantro, lemon juice and zest, then toss them all to coat evenly. Serve the prawns with arugula and crusty bread.

20. Buffalo Chicken Burgers

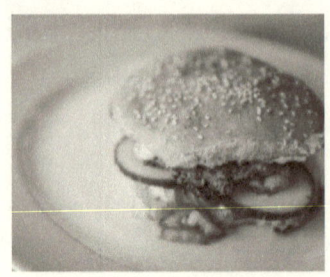

For 4 burgers

Put a smile on everyone's face with these scrumptious chicken burgers.

Ingredients

- 2 Tbsps. of Butter
- ½ a cup of Buffalo Sauce
- 3 cups of Shredded Rotisserie Chicken
- 1 small cucumber, sliced in rings
- 4 Whole Grain Buns (toasted)
- 4 oz. of Blue Cheese (crumbled)
- Celery Stalks to serve

Method

1. Toast the whole grain buns. Melt the butter in a pan over a medium heat; add the buffalo sauce and the chicken. Cook this mixture for 2-4 minutes, stirring occasionally.

2. Place the cucumber rings on the toasted bun base and then divide the cooked chicken mixture evenly among the buns. Sprinkle on the blue cheese and place the toasted tops on the buns and serve with celery stalks.

21. Quick Falafels

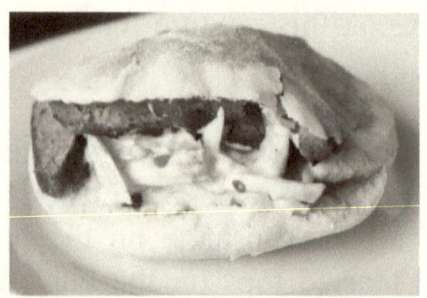

Makes 4 Falafels

Change up the menu with these healthy and scrumptious falafels.

Ingredients

- ¼ of a cup of Minced Red Onion
- 1 Tbsp. of Dijon Mustard
- 1 tsp of Ground Cumin
- 1 tsp of Paprika
- ½ a tsp of Pepper
- 1/8 of a tsp of Salt
- 1 (15.5oz.) can of Chickpeas (drained)
- 1 slice Whole Grain Bread (torn into pieces)

- 2 large Eggs

- 2 Tbsps. of Olive Oil

- 4 Whole Grain Pitas

- 1 cup of Arugula

- ½ a cup of Tzatziki Sauce (chilled)

Method

1. In a food processor, pulse together the first 9 ingredients on the list until they are well blended. Heat the oil in a pan over medium to high heat. Divide the chickpea mixture into 1/3 cup portions/balls.

2. Drop each portion into the hot pan and cook for 4 minutes each side. Divide the arugula evenly among pitas and add 1 falafel ball into each. Then spoon in Tzatziki sauce and serve.

22. Veggie Chili with Salad

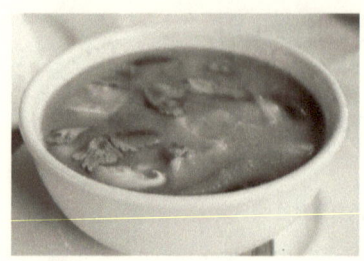

Makes enough for 4 servings

This chili may not have any meat, but it's still just as hearty and satisfying.

Ingredients

- 1 Dried, Smoked Chili (chopped)
- 2 Fresh Red Chilies (chopped, divided)
- 1 Red Onion (halved)
- 1 tsp of Paprika
- ½ a tsp of Cumin Seeds
- 2 Garlic Cloves (crushed)
- 1 bunch of Fresh Cilantro (leaves and stalks separated)
- 2 Bell Peppers

- 1 lb. of canned Black Beans (drained)
- 1 lb. of canned Chickpeas (drained)
- 3 cups of Tomato Paste
- ¼ of a lb. of Cooked Wild Rice
- 4 small Corn Tortillas (sliced into strips)
- 2 Avocados (peeled, chopped)
- 3 Tbsps. of Plain Greek Yogurt (plus extra)
- 2 Limes
- 1 head of Romaine Lettuce (cut in wedges)
- ½ a cucumber (sliced into ribbons)
- 1 handful of Cherry Tomatoes (halved)
- Olive Oil as needed

Method

1. In a processor, pulse together the onion, garlic, paprika, cumin seeds, smoked chili, and 1 fresh chili. Add the cilantro stalks and 2 tablespoons olive oil. Blending the mixture until it's finely minced.

2. Add the mixture to a pan on high heat with the remaining fresh chili, chickpeas, and black beans. Add salt and pepper to taste, then stir in the tomato paste until well mixed. Cover the mixture and allow it to cook.

3. Arrange the tortilla strips on a baking sheet and bake them in a preheated oven at 400°F, until they are golden brown. Then remove them and set them aside in a bowl.

4. In the food processor, pulse together half the avocado, the yogurt, cilantro leaves, lime juice, salt and pepper until the mixture is silky smooth.

5. Place the lettuce in the bowl with the tortilla strips and spoon in the remaining avocado and cucumber. Pour the rice into the chili mixture, cover it and let cook 2-3 minutes.

6. Pour the avocado-lime mixture over the lettuce-tortilla salad, add the tomatoes and toss it all together to combine. Serve the chili with dollops of yogurt and the salad alongside.

23. Fried Rice and Eggs

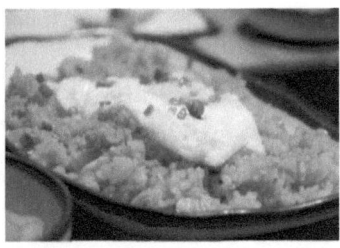

Makes enough for 4 servings

The whole family will love this surprisingly healthy recipe

Ingredients

- 2 Tbsps. of Rice Bran Oil
- 2 Garlic Cloves (minced)
- 1 Fresh Red Chili (chopped)
- 2 tsp. of Grated Ginger
- 1 cup of Snow Peas (sliced)
- 4 cups of Brown Rice (cooked)
- 1 tsp of Powdered Sugar
- 2 tsp of Fish Sauce
- 2 Tbsps. of Low Sodium Soy Sauce

- 1/3 of a cup of Unsalted Roasted Peanuts (chopped)

- 4 Eggs

- 1 Tbsp. of Shichimi (a Japanese spice mix)

Method

1. Heat 1 Tbsp of the oil in a wok over a medium to high heat. Stir-fry the garlic, chili and ginger for 15 seconds, then add the snow peas, stir-frying for 1 minute. Then add the rice, stir-fry another minute and add the peanuts, sugar, soy sauce, and fish sauce. Stir-fry this for an additional minute, then remove it from the heat and set it aside.

2. In a separate pan, heat the remaining oil over medium to high heat. Crack the eggs into the pan and cook them to your preferred degree/taste.

3. Divide the rice mixture into 4 bowls and top each with 1 egg, then sprinkle them with the shichimi mix and serve.

24. Buttermilk Chicken Salad

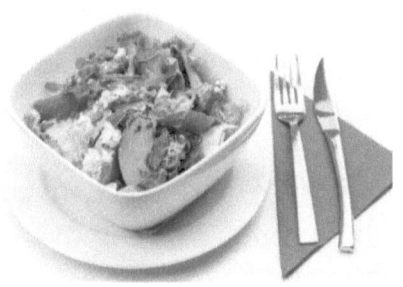

Makes 4 servings

This quick and scrumptious salad makes for the perfect lunch.

Ingredients

- ¼ of a cup of Buttermilk
- ¼ of a cup of Mayonnaise
- 1 Tbsp. of Fresh Lemon Juice
- 4 Plum Tomatoes (chopped)
- 2 Romaine Lettuce Hearts (torn into small pieces)
- 1 (2-2.5 lbs.) Rotisserie Chicken (chopped)
- ½ a Tbsp. of Fresh Chives (chopped)
- Salt & Pepper to taste

Method

1. In a bowl, whisk together the buttermilk, mayonnaise and lemon juice, add the tomatoes with salt and pepper to taste.

2. Divide the lettuce and chicken among plates and spoon the buttermilk dressing over the top. Sprinkle them with the chives and serve.

25. Portobello Mushroom Salad

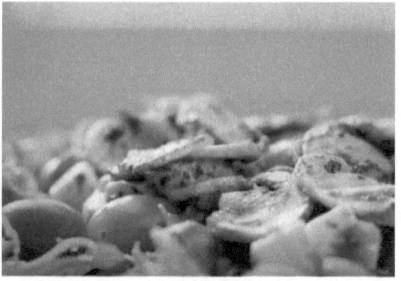

Makes 4 servings

This quick salad is perfect for a nice dinner party or a regular family dinner night.

Ingredients

- ¼ of a cup of Red Wine Vinegar
- ¼ of a cup of Balsamic Vinegar
- ¼ of a cup of Tomato Juice
- Olive Oil as needed
- 2 tsp of Dijon Mustard
- 2 tsp of Stoneground Mustard
- 4 large Portobello Mushroom Tops
- 1 Tbsp. of Cajun Steak Seasoning

- 4 cups of fresh Salad Greens

- 1 Tomato (cut into 8 wedges)

- 1 Red Onion (sliced)

- 1 cup of canned White Beans (drained)

- 4 Tbsps. of Crumbled Blue Cheese

Method

1. Combine the first 7 ingredients on the list, in a large re-sealable bag and shake it so they are well mixed. Add the mushrooms and allow them to marinate in the liquid for 10 minutes. Then remove the mushrooms and sprinkle them with Cajun seasoning and set the marinade aside.

2. Heat the oil in a large pan over a medium to high heat and saute the mushrooms for 2 minutes each side, then allow them to cool slightly before slicing.

3. Place a cup of salad greens on each plate and top this with the sliced mushrooms, tomato wedges, and onion. Add a ¼ of a cup of beans and 1 Tbsp of blue cheese to each plate. Drizzle the marinade over each salad and serve.

26. Beef Kofta on Rice

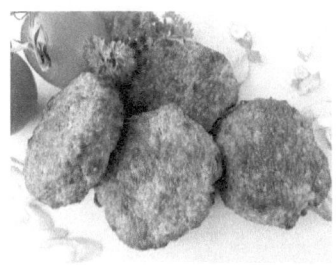

Servings enough for 4 people

Spice up your dinner table with this variation on the classic Indian dish.

Ingredients

- ¼ of a lb. of Red Lentils
- 1 tsp of Garam Masala
- 1 lb. of Ground Beef
- 3 Tomatoes
- 1 (2") piece of Ginger (grated)
- 2 Spring Onions
- 1 bunch of Fresh Cilantro
- 1 Fresh Red Chili

- 1 tsp of Turmeric
- 1 tsp of Honey
- 2 tsp of Curry Paste
- 1 cup of Coconut Milk
- 1 Lemon
- 1 cup of Brown Rice (cooked)
- 5 Cardamom Pods
- 1 cup of Green Beans
- 1 cup of Frozen Peas
- Olive Oil as needed
- Plain Greek Yogurt to serve

Method

1. In a food processor, quickly pulse together the lentils, beef, garam masala, salt and pepper until they are just combined. Divide the mixture into 12 equal portions and shape them into long roll shapes or balls (like large meat balls).

2. Fry the lentil rolls in a pan over a high heat with 1 tablespoon oil until they are golden brown all over.

Arrange the cardamom pods in a pan or casserole dish with the green beans.

3. In a food processor, pulse together the tomatoes, ginger, spring onions, half the chili, cilantro stalks, honey, coconut milk, turmeric, and curry paste. Then pour this into the pan with the lentils. Bring this mixture to the boil, then reduce the heat to a medium simmer.

4. Add the peas to the rice and cook these over a medium heat until cooked through. Sprinkle the cilantro leaves and remaining chili over the Kofta. Serve the Kofta with a dollop of yogurt and lemon wedges on top of the rice and green beans.

27. Lemon Tuna Pasta

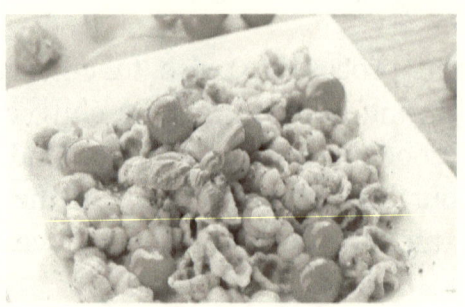

Makes enough for 4 people

Ingredients

- 1 lb. of Short Pasta (cooked)
- 1 ½ Tbsps. Of Capers (drained)
- 1 cup of Fresh Parsley
- 1 cup of Fresh Basil
- 1 Garlic Clove (chopped)
- 2 Anchovy Fillets
- 1 tsp of Dijon Mustard
- Zest and Juice of 1 Lemon
- 1 lb. of canned Tuna (drained, but retain the oil)

- A handful of small cherry tomatoes for a garnish

Method

1. Pat the capers dry with a paper towel and place 2 tsp of them in a food processor or blender together with the anchovies, garlic, mustard, herbs, lemon juice and zest, then pulse them a few times until they are coarsely chopped.

2. Drizzle in the tuna oil while still pulsing until mixture becomes a coarse paste. Stir this paste into the pasta until evenly coated, then stir in the tuna and remaining capers, stirring until well combined.

3. Serve with the whole cherry tomatoes and fresh small basil leaves.

28. Ravioli Zucchini Sauté

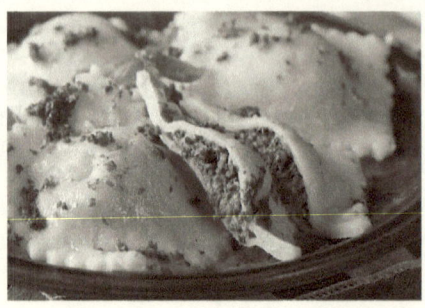

Makes 2 portions

Cheesy ravioli is upgraded with zucchini and Parmesan in this delicious but quick recipe.

Ingredients

- 1 lb. of Cheese Ravioli (cooked)
- 2 Tbsps. of Olive Oil
- 3 small Zucchini (sliced)
- 2 Garlic Cloves (sliced)
- ½ a cup of Grated Parmesan
- Salt & Pepper to taste

Method

1. Heat the oil in a large pan over a medium heat, then add the sliced zucchini and season with salt and pepper to taste.

2. Cook this mixture for 4-5 minutes, stirring occasionally, then add the garlic and cook for a further 2 minutes, stirring often.

3. Add the zucchini mixture and ¼ of a cup of Parmesan to the ravioli and toss it well to combine. Then serve it with the remaining Parmesan sprinkled on top.

29. Almond Kale Salad

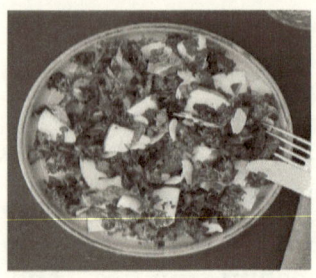

Serves 2 portions

This ultra-healthy dish is surprisingly delicious and pairs perfectly with the lamb burgers found earlier in this book.

Ingredients

- 2 Tbsps. of Minced Shallots
- 1 ½ Tbsps. of Olive Oil
- 2 tsp of Fresh Lemon Juice
- 2 tsp of Dijon Mustard
- ¼ of a tsp of Pepper
- 1/8 of a tsp of Salt
- 1 Garlic Clove
- ½ a lb. of Brussels Sprouts (thinly sliced)

- ¼ of a cup of Sliced Almonds
- 1 cup of Chopped Kale
- 1 small Red Apple (thinly sliced)
- 2 Tbsps. Of Parmesan

Method

1. In a small bowl, stir together the first 7 ingredients on the list, to make the dressing.
2. In a large bowl, toss together the kale, Brussels sprouts, and almonds, then add the dressing to the kale mixture and toss the salad before sprinkling it with the Parmesan cheese.

30. Stuffed Quesadillas

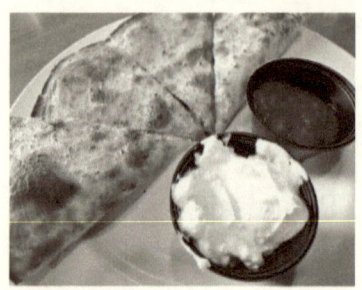

Enough for 4 people

Increase the nutritional value and the taste of quesadillas with this easy recipe.

Ingredients

- 1 (15.5oz.) can of Black Beans (drained)
- 1 (11oz.) can of Corn (drained)
- ¾ of a cup of Salsa
- 8 large Flour Tortillas
- 1 ½ cups of Grated Cheddar Cheese
- 1 Red Onion (sliced)
- 1/3 of a cup of Fresh Cilantro
- 1-2 limes (juiced)

- 2 Tbsps. of Olive Oil

- 1 head of Romaine Lettuce (cut into 1" strips)

- Salt & Pepper to taste

Method

1. Preheat your oven to 400°F. In a bowl, mix together the corn, beans, and salsa. Place 4 tortillas on a baking sheet lined with parchment paper.

2. Sprinkle ¾ of a cup of cheese over the tortillas and top them with the bean mixture. Then place the remaining tortillas on top. Sprinkle the remaining cheese over the top of these and bake this for 5-7 minutes.

3. In another bowl, combine cilantro, onion, lime juice, oil, salt and pepper. Add the lettuce and toss it well to coat it all evenly and serve the salad alongside the quesadillas.

31. Pork Tofu Stir-Fry

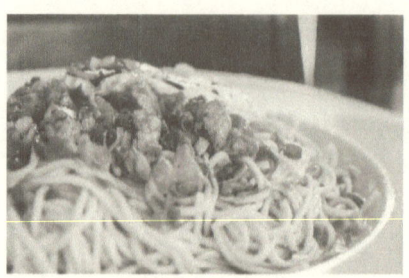

Enough for 4 servings

Silky tofu and juicy pork, combine well together in this perfect stir-fry dish.

Ingredients

- 2 tsp of Corn Flour
- ½ a cup of Chicken Stock
- 1 Tbsp. of Rice Wine
- 1 lb. of Ground Pork
- 1 ½ Tbsps. of Hoisin Sauce
- 3 Garlic Cloves (crushed)
- 1 (1") piece of Ginger (grated)
- 1 lb. of Firm Tofu (cubed)

- 2 Green Onions (sliced)

- 1 Fresh Red Chili (minced)

- Fresh butter noodles or Steamed Jasmine Rice to serve

Method

1. In a jug, stir together the cornflour, wine, and stock until they are well blended. Place a little oil in a wok and put it over a high heat, then quickly add the ground pork and stir-fry this for 3 minutes.

2. Add the garlic, chili, ginger, and hoisin sauce to the wok and stir in the stock mixture from the jug. Bring the mixture to the boil and add the tofu. Reduce the heat and simmer it for 2 minutes. Then serve the stir-fry over noodles or rice, topped with the green onions.

32. Tuna Bean Salad

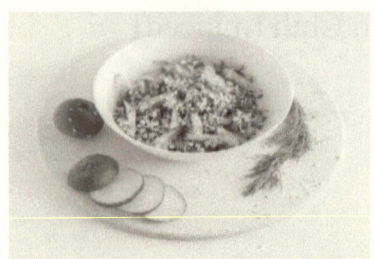

Makes 4 servings

This simple salad makes for an effortlessly satisfying lunch.

Ingredients

- ¼ of a cup of Olive Oil
- 3 Tbsps. of Fresh Lemon Juice
- 3 cups of Torn Basil Leaves
- 1 bulb of Fennel (thinly sliced)
- ¼ of a cup of Chopped Fennel Fronds
- 2 (6oz.) cans of Tuna (drained)
- 1 (15.5oz.) can of White Beans (drained)
- 1 Shallot (thinly sliced)

- Salt & Pepper to taste

Method

1. In a large bowl, whisk together the lemon juice, oil, salt and pepper. Add remaining ingredients and toss to combine, allow the dressing to infuse for a few minutes then serve.

33. Tarragon Chicken

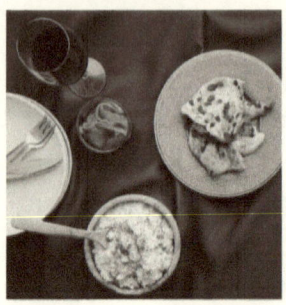

Makes 4 servings

Spice up the classic chicken dinner with this bold recipe.

Ingredients

- 4 (6oz.) Skinless Boneless Chicken Breasts
- ¼ of a tsp Salt
- 2 Tbsps. of Olive Oil
- 1 tsp of Lemon Zest
- 1 Garlic Clove (minced)
- 2 tsp of Minced Tarragon
- 1/8 of tsp of Salt

Method

1. Fold the chicken breasts in parchment paper and pound them with a mallet until they are ¼" thick. Sprinkle a ¼ of a tsp of salt evenly over all breasts. Whisk together remaining 5 ingredients in a small bowl to make a seasoned oil.

2. Heat a pan over medium to high heat and add 2 tsp of the seasoned oil to coat pan, then add the chicken. Cook it for 2 minutes and drizzle 2 teaspoons oil mixture over chicken, turn it over and cook other side for 2 minutes.

3. Drizzle the rest of the oil mixture over the chicken. Reduce the heat to low and cover it, continue cooking the chicken for 2 minutes longer, then remove it from the heat. Arrange the chicken on a platter. Drizzle the pan drippings over the top and serve it with rice or fresh salad.

34. Spaghetti with Fresh Tomato Sauce and Basil Leaves

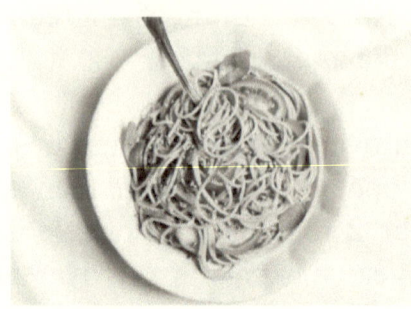

Enough for 4 servings

A Quick and tasty vegetarian spaghetti made with fresh tomatoes to make a clean, wholesome and tasty sauce, then garnished with tomato wedges, basil leaves and shaved Parmesan Cheese.

Ingredients

- 1 lb of fresh, juicy, ripe Tomatoes, sliced in half
- 1 small Onion, diced
- 2 cloves of Garlic, diced
- 2 tsp of fresh Lime Juice
- 1 tbsp of Virgin Olive Oil
- 12 to 14 ounces of Spaghetti

- 1 tsp of Italian Seasoning

- Sea salt and freshly cracked Black Pepper to taste

- A few fresh Basil Leaves

- Freshly shaved Parmesan Cheese

Method

1. Cook the Pasta according to the instructions on the packet to "Al dente" about 10 to 12 minutes. While the pasta is cooking, take 2 of the nicest looking tomatoes and slice them into wedges.

2. Place the rest of the tomatoes in a pressure cooker with the garlic, onion, Italian seasoning, salt and pepper and cook for 10 minutes. Remove the Tomatoes from the pressure cooker and blend them in a food processor or blender until smooth.

3. Pass the sauce through a fine sieve to remove the seeds and skins (optional). Add the lime juice and olive oil and adjust the seasoning to taste by adding extra salt and pepper if required.

4. Drain the pasta in a colander the while still hot, place it in a serving dish and stir in the sauce. Add the tomato wedges and basil leaves and allow the pasta flavors to infuse for a few minutes, then serve with the shaved Parmesan on top.

35. Sea Bream Baked with Rosemary and Lemon

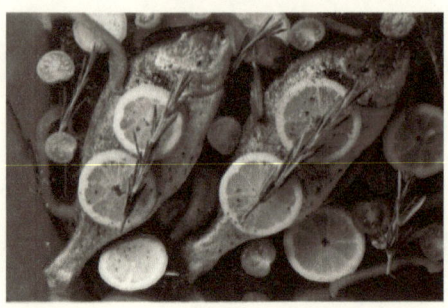

Enough for 2 servings

Sea bream is a very tasty and sweet fleshed fish, it is well matched with lemon and rosemary, the combination brings a lovely freshness to the meal

Ingredients

- 2 whole, plate sized Sea Bream
- A large Lemon cut into Rings
- 4 sprigs of Fresh Rosemary
- 2 or 3 Tomatoes, sliced in thick rings
- 4 to 6 tbsp of Olive or Coconut Oil
- Sea Salt and freshly cracked Black Pepper to taste

Method

1. Heat your oven to a high heat about 420F (220C). Wash the fish and carefully remove the insides, chop off the fins and pat the fish dry using a paper towel.

2. Rub the body cavity with a little sea salt, before placing a few lemon rings and a sprig of rosemary inside the fish. Brush the outside with Oil and arrange the rest of the lemon the tomato rings and rosemary on and around the fish and in an additional dish.

3. Place the fish on a wire rack over a baking dish to catch any juices. Bake for 12 to 14 minutes or until the flesh is only just cooked, do not over cook. Serve with the cooked lemon, tomato and rosemary on rice and accompanied by your favorite salad.

36. Brown Onion and Garlic Soup with Sour Cream

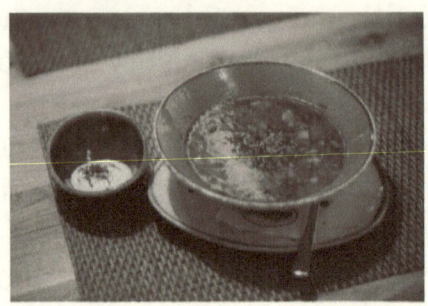

Enough for 8 cups

This delicious Onion and Garlic soup is thickened with bread, the same way as traditionally done in the South of France, to give a warm satisfying and filling soup.

Ingredients

- 7 cups of Stock or Broth either Beef, Chicken or Vegetable

- 3 large Onions

- 12 cloves of Garlic

- 3 tbsp of Olive or Coconut Oil

- 6 slices of your favorite bread (whole grain or white)

- Sea Salt and freshly cracked Black Pepper to taste

- 1 Spring Onion (Green Onion)

- ½ a cup of Sour Cream

Method

1. Heat the broth either in a microwave or large stockpot on your stove top. Place a large, heavy bottomed saucepan containing the 3 tbsp of oil on a medium heat. While the oil is heating, peel and chop the onion roughly.

2. Saute the onions, stirring while you peel and chop the garlic roughly then add them to the onions. Allow the onions and garlic to soften, about 5 minutes, then add the hot stock and simmer covered for 5 minutes.

3. Dice the bread into about ½ inch cubes a place these into the soup. Slice the spring onions, finely as a garnish and set them aside.

4. When the bread has softened and absorbed the soup. Place ¾ of the mixture in a blender and puree it until smooth, then return this to the saucepan for a chunky textured soup or if preferred, puree it all for a smooth soup. Taste the soup and add salt and pepper as required and then serve in bowls with a little sour cream and spring onions.

37. Pressure Cooker Chicken with Orange

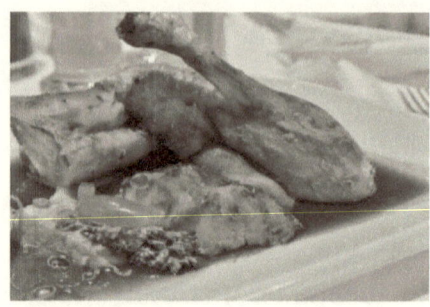

Serves 2 generous portions

This healthy fast method of cooking chicken ensures it is moist, tender and full of flavor. As a bonus, you also get a rich gravy or sauce that can be thickened with a little rice flour or arrowroot to add the final touch to your meal. If you do not have a pressure cooker this recipe will take about an hour in a saucepan on the stove top.

Ingredients

- 1 whole Chicken or 4 large Chicken Legs
- 1 cup of Chicken Stock
- 1/2 a cup of fresh Orange Juice
- 1 medium Onion, diced
- 2 cloves of Garlic, minced
- 1 tbsp of Oyster Sauce

- A Bouquet garni made with 1 Basil Leaf, 3 springs of Parsley, 1 sprig of Thyme and an optional sprig of Rosemary (or use a little of your favorite herbs, dried or fresh)

- 1 large Sweet Potato cut into bite sized pieces

- Sea Salt and freshly cracked Black Pepper to taste

- 1 to 2 tbsp of Rice Flour

Method

1. Place all the liquid ingredients in your pressure cooker with the bouquet garni onion and garlic, and then put the cooking tray in place to keep the chicken above the level of the liquid.

2. Sprinkle salt and pepper over the chicken and then place it with the sweet potato in the cooking baskets or on top of the cooking tray and shut the lid. Cook the chicken at full heat for 10 minutes, then allow to cool so you can safely open and remove the chicken and sweet potato.

3. Taste the gravy and add more salt and Pepper to taste. (Sweet potatoes absorb a lot of salt). Add rice flour to a very small amount of water, then stir this into the gravy to thicken and simmer of about a minute before serving it either over the chicken or on a gravy boat alongside.

38. Thai Seafood Curry with Egg Noodles

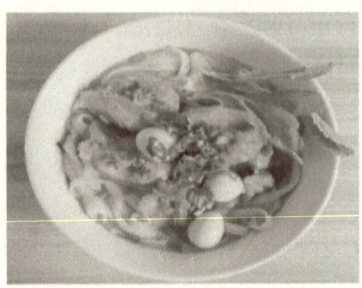

Enough for 4 servings

This spicy seafood soup is quick and easy to make and will impress even the most discerning diners with its crisp clean taste and pallet pleasing flavors.

Ingredients

- 8 to 12 large peeled Prawns

- 8 to 12 whole Scallops

- 1 medium Squid Tube sliced into thin rings

- 150g of fresh Fish, Salmon, Grouper or Cod etc. diced into ½ to ¾ inch cubes

- 2 cloves of Garlic, finely diced

- 1 small piece of Ginger Finely sliced

- 1 small Onion, thinly sliced

- 1 to 2 tbsp of Red Thai Curry Paste (more if you like it hot)

- 1 tsp of Fish Sauce

- 1 cup of Coconut Cream

- The Juice of 1 Lime

- A small handful of fresh Coriander, roughly chopped

- 1 Spring Onion for the garnish

- 2 tbsp of finely sliced Red Capsicum (Pepper) for the garnish

- Sea Salt and Black Pepper to taste

- 2 tbsp of Coconut Oil

- 1 tsp of Sesame Oil

- ½ a cup of fresh Water

- One packet of instant Egg Noodles

Method

1. Place the noodles in a large saucepan of boiling, salted water for 2 minutes, then drain and refresh them (cool in cold water). Place the coconut and

sesame oils in a wok or large frying pan and bring them to a medium heat.

2. Saute the onion, ginger and garlic until they soften, about 2 minutes while constantly stirring. Add the curry paste, fish sauce, coconut cream and lime juice, then stir this mixture to combine.

3. Add the fish, scallops, prawns and squid and cook for about 3 minutes. If the mixture is too dry and there is not much sauce add the water. Then stir in the coriander and serve on the cool noodles.

39. Baked Pizza Rolls

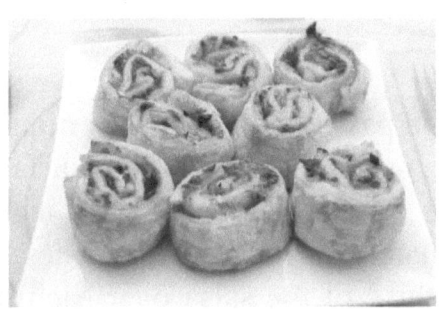

Serves 4 people

A quick, tasty alternative to making a baked lasagne, they go well with a light salad for a substantial meal and can be eaten hot or cold so make a great school or office lunch. You can also add any preferred items such as olives, mushrooms, chili, ground beef, chicken or seafoods.

Ingredients

- 1 x 8 ounce pack of Flaky Pastry

- ½ a cup of Tomato Sauce

- 1 cup of grated Mozzarella or Tasty Cheddar Cheese

- ½ a cup of finely sliced Ham

- Several Bok Choy or Chinese Cabbage Leaves Finely shredded

- 1 tbsp of Italian or Pizza Spices

- Any other desired additions

Method

1. Divide the pastry into 3 equal portions and roll each one out on a clean, floured surface to form a rectangle about 1/8 of an inch thick and approximately 14 inches by 8 inches. Evenly spread about a third of the salsa over each piece of rolled out pastry.

2. Add a thin layer of cheese, a layer of ham and a layer of shredded Bok choy as well as any extras you wish to add. Give a generous sprinkle of spices.

3. Roll the long side over several times so it forms a tight cylinder, then slice it into 12 even slices. Place the slices on a well-oiled baking tray and bake them in a preheated oven at 400f (200C) for about 10 minutes.

40. Super Fast Pizza

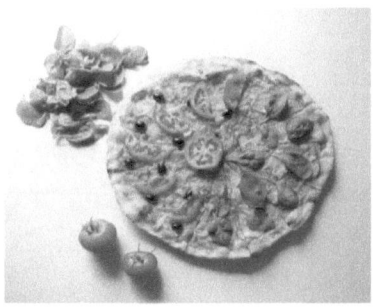

6 individual pizzas

These pizzas use a toasted pita bread base with fresh tomato salsa, mozzarella cheese and any other ingredients you have at hand. They are great for a quick lunch at home or work for all members of the family to enjoy.

Ingredients

- 6 x 8 inch Fresh Toasted Pita Bread

- 1½ cups of Tomato Salsa

- 1 cup of grated Mozzarella Cheese

- 1 cup of grated Edam or other Cheese you like

- 1 tbsp of Italian or Pizza Spices

- Any desired additions, some suggestions are: Ham, Bacon, Chicken or Seafood's, Tomato, Onion,

Capsicum, Olives, Mushroom, Herbs and vegetables or fruit such as Pineapple, Mango or Avocados

Method

1. Have your oven very hot at 450F (225C). Place the toasted pita bread on a baking tray. Cover the top with a layer of tomato salsa. Add your chosen toppings.

2. Sprinkle on a generous amount of cheese and pizza spice. Bake for 10 minutes. Serve while hot or keep and serve cold as a delicious snack.

Final Words

I would like to thank you for downloading my book and I hope I have been able to help you and educate you about something new.

If you have enjoyed this book and would like to share your positive thoughts, could you please take 30 seconds of your time to go back and give me a review on my Amazon book page!

I greatly appreciate seeing these reviews because it helps me share my hard work!

Again, thank you and I wish you all the best with your cooking journey!

Last Chance to Get YOUR Bonus!

FOR A LIMITED TIME ONLY – Get Olivia's best-selling book *"The #1 Cookbook: Over 170+ of the Most Popular Recipes Across 7 Different Cuisines!"* absolutely FREE!

Readers have absolutely loved this book because of the wide variety of recipes. It is highly recommended you check these recipes out and see what you can add to your home menu!

Once again, as a big thank-you for downloading this book, I'd like to offer it to you *100% FREE for a LIMITED TIME ONLY!*

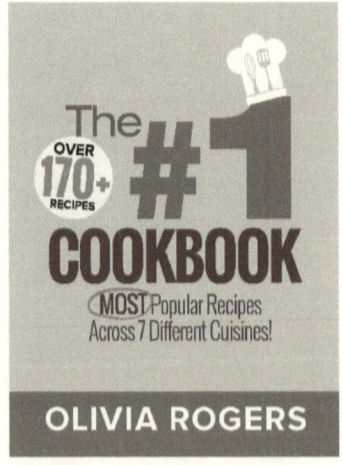

Get your free copy at:

TheMenuAtHome.com/Bonus

Disclaimer

This book and related site provides recipe and food advice in an informative and educational manner only, with information that is general in nature and that is not specific to you, the reader. The contents of this book and related site are intended to assist you and other readers in your personal efforts. Consult your physician or nutritionist regarding the applicability of any information provided in our information to you.

Nothing in this book should be construed as personal advice or diagnosis, and must not be used in this manner. The information provided about conditions is general in nature. This information does not cover all possible uses, actions, precautions, side-effects, or interactions of medicines, or medical procedures. The information in this site should not be considered as complete and does not cover all diseases, ailments, physical conditions, or their treatment.

No Warranties: The authors and publishers don't guarantee or warrant the quality, accuracy, completeness, timeliness, appropriateness or suitability of the information in this book, or of any product or services referenced by this site.

The information in this site is provided on an "as is" basis and the authors and publishers make no representations or warranties of any kind with respect to this information. This site may contain inaccuracies, typographical errors, or other errors.

Liability Disclaimer: The publishers, authors, and other parties involved in the creation, production, provision of information, or delivery of this site specifically disclaim any responsibility, and shall not be held liable for any damages, claims, injuries, losses, liabilities, costs, or obligations including any direct, indirect, special, incidental, or consequences damages (collectively known as "Damages") whatsoever and howsoever caused, arising out of, or in connection with the use or misuse of the site and the information contained within it, whether such Damages arise in contract, tort, negligence, equity, statute law, or by way of other legal theory.

www.ingramcontent.com/pod-product-compliance
Lightning Source LLC
Chambersburg PA
CBHW021128080526
44587CB00012B/1184